# MENTAL HEALTH AND DIET

## *HOW TO EAT WITH YOUR MENTAL HEALTH IN MIND*

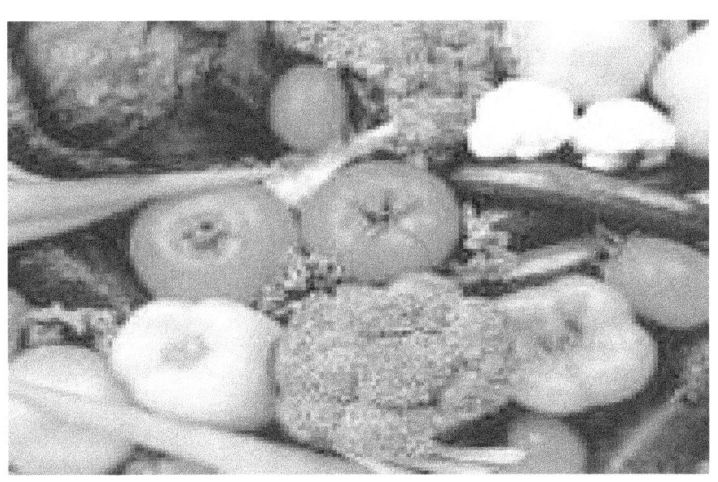

### By Patricia A. Carlisle

# Introduction

I want to thank you and congratulate you for choosing the book, *"MENTAL HEALTH AND DIET: How to Eat with Your Mental Health in Mind"*.

This book contains proven steps and strategies on how good nutrition is essential for our mental health.

Recent studies recommend that good nutrition is essential for our mental health, and that various mental health conditions may be affected by dietary factors. A standout amongst the most self-evident, yet under-perceived factors in the advancement of major patterns in mental health is the part of nutrition. The body of evidence connecting eating routine, and mental health is developing at a rapid pace. As well as its impact on short and long haul towards mental health, the confirmation proof that food plays an important contributing part in the advancement, management and avoidance of particular mental health issues, for example, sadness, schizophrenia, attention deficiency hyperactivity issue, and Alzheimer's disease.

Thanks again for choosing this book, I hope you enjoy it!

# ABOUT THE AUTHOR
# PATRICIA A. CARLISLE, MSW, CBT

Patricia Carlisle- a Master Social Worker and Cognitive Behavioral Therapist (CBT) gives out an expression of how important it is for an individual to take into consideration the concept of self-assessment to know what human, technical and conceptual skills they posses to perform or to achieve what they desire, or to deal with everyday life. However, every particular group of people has their own unique set of ideas, traditions and events including the frame of mind according to which people perform but there are many who faces problems and fail to maintain a healthy mind set affecting their behaviors and performance to those around them.

*People like Patricia Carlisle are among those who have felt this urge of serving people and helping them out of their mental crisis towards a healthy life. She has experienced some close encounters in her personal life regarding mental health issues in her family and friends that has encouraged her to pursue this as her career.*

Currently Patricia Carlisle is serving as a Certified On-Line Cognitive Behavioral Therapist with an extensive 15years of experience using Cognitive-Behavior Therapy Techniques. She envisions a world where everyone gets mental health treatment with no mental health stigma and to make it real she has already set up her own Holistic Measure Online Comprehensive Behavioral Healthcare Company after retiring from The Nord Center in The Partial Hospitalization Program (PHP) Dept for 5 years and Murtis H. Taylor Mental Health Center as a mental health counselor, psychological support technician and case manager for 10 years to emulsify her skills more professionally.

Along with this, she has wrote down her passion as a clinician in 25 or more short books to help individuals and families get their life back, freeing them of the restraints of negative thinking, anxiety and depression by using different approaches. She is highly appreciated among her clients for her flexibility and professionalism of dealing with them graciously. To reach her, make use of her direct website address: http://therapist2013.wix.com/e-therapy . As she is ready to inspire hope and contribute to health and well-being by providing the best online health care through comprehensive practice, education and research.

# TABLE OF CONTENT

# Chapter 9

## DIETARY SUPPLEMENTS

### Preview of 'JUICING TO HELP MENTAL ILLNESS'

# Chapter 1

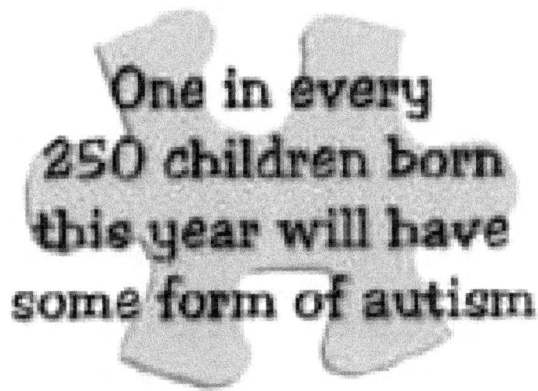

One in every
250 children born
this year will have
some form of autism

## MENTAL HEALTH AND DIET STATISTICS

Nearly 66% of the individuals who don't report daily mental health issues eat fresh organic product or organic product squeeze consistently, compared with not as much as half of the individuals who do report daily mental health issues. This pattern is similar for fresh vegetables and salad. The individuals who report some level of mental health issue also eat less healthy foods (fresh foods grown from the ground, organic foods, and meals made from scratch), and more unhealthy food (chips and crisps, chocolate, ready meals, and takeaways).

A balance disposition and emotions of wellbeing can be secured by guaranteeing that our eating routine gives adequate amounts of complex carbohydrates, essential fats, amino acids, vitamins and minerals and water. While a healthy eating routine can help recuperation, it should sit alongside different treatments suggested by your specialist.

What we are eating now is altogether different from that of our recent ancestors. Food generation and manufacturing methods, combined with changing ways of life and increasing access to processed foods, mean that our intake of fresh, nutritious, local produce is much lower, at the same time as our intake of fat, sugar, alcohol and additives is much higher. It has been estimated that the average individual in the US, and other industrialized nations will eat more than 4 kilograms or 4000 grams of additives consistently.

Throughout the last 60 years there has been a 34% decrease in US vegetable utilization with as of now just 13% of men, and 15% of women now eating at least five parts of products of the soil every day. Individuals in the UK eat 59% less fish than they did 60 years ago-decreasing the utilization of essential omega-3fatty acids. A healthy eating routine can be more extravagant. Fish, foods grown from the ground can be particularly pricey.

On the other hand, by eliminating sugary beverages and snacks, and taking a way alcohol, you can save money, and you would be able to purchase healthier foods. Take care to purchase what you can use to diminish waste.

# Chapter 2

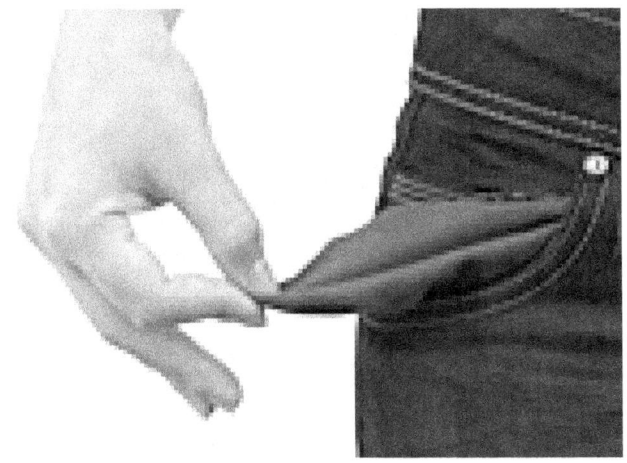

## HOW TO CUT YOUR FOOD EXPENSES

You can also cut your expenses by taking advantage of special advancements, and by shopping at market stands, which are cheaper than supermarkets. If you live alone you could save cash by purchasing with companions (purchasing mass is usually cheaper), or by cooking small dishes and freezing some of them. This also saves you the time of preparing meals consistently.

Solidified foods grown from the ground are often cheaper than fresh deliver, and have a greater nutritionally with no wastage. Fresh leafy foods are usually cheapest when they are in season. Beans, lentils and soy mince are also cheaper than meat and generally as nutritious. Eat regular meals for the duration of the day to maintain glucose levels.

Make sure beyond any doubt you eat at least three meals each day. Missing meals, especially breakfast, leads to low glucose, and this causes low mind-set, irritability and fatigue. If you feel hungry between meals you may need to incorporate a healthy snack for instance, a natural product, nuts and cereals.

Eat less, high sugar foods and more wholegrain oats, nuts, beans, lentils, foods grown from the ground. Sugary foods are assimilated rapidly into the circulation system. This may bring about a starting "high", or surge of vitality that soon wears off as the body builds its insulin generation, abandoning you feeling drained and tired.

# Chapter 3

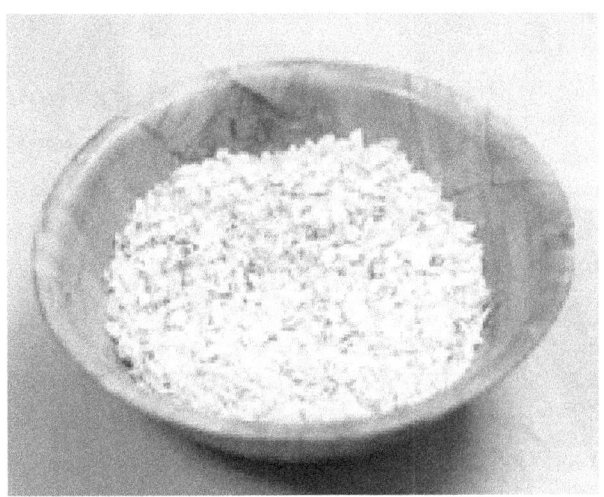

## FOODS THAT DON'T BRING ABOUT EMOTIONAL EPISODES

Wholegrain oats, and foods grown from the ground are additionally filling, and in light of the fact that the sugar in these foods are consumed all the more gradually don't bring about emotional episodes. These foods are not nutritious as they contain thiamin, a vitamin that has been connected with controlling your state of mind, and foliate and zinc. Supplements of these nutrients has been demonstrated to enhance the disposition of individuals with depression.

1. **Bread**-Brown instead of white. Likewise, tend Rye breads, pumpernickel, oat cakes, rice cakes and corn cakes.

2. **Breakfast** -oats-pick high fiver, low sugar such as wholegrain or grain oats or porridge.

3. **Rice and pasta**-go for Basmati, coca rice which gives a nutty composition in serving of mixed greens, and wholegrain pasta.

4. **Potatoes**-serve boiled and in their skins (with a little margarine) or squashed potatoes, Potato wedges (delicately brushed with olive oil) are a lower fat option for chips and meal potatoes if you are watching your weight. Attempt sweet potatoes or yams for a change-these are heavenly prepared.

Try to eat no less than five segments of vegetables and fruits a day for instance, 1 glass of squeezed orange or ½ grapefruit for breakfast, a banana or apple for brunch, a plate of mixed greens at lunch time, and after that two types of vegetable (two serving).

# Chapter 4

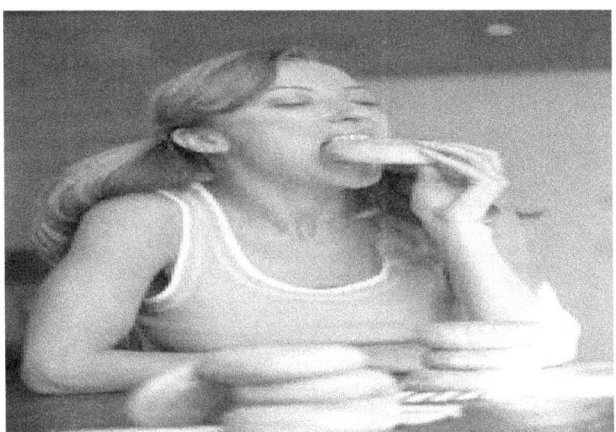

## FOODS TO KEEP AWAY FROM

Keep away from sugar and sugary beverages, cakes, deserts and puddings. These are stacked with calories and have minimal nourishing quality, and may trigger emotional episodes because of the high amount of sugar content.

Incorporate protein at each meal to guarantee a large amount of the amino corrosive tryptophan to the brain. Eating a well balance amount of protein will help keep our skin, organs, muscle healthy. Late research proposes that one specific part of protein, (the amino corrosive tryptophan), can have a high impact on your state of mind.

Supplements of tryptophan were tried in studies, and some were demonstrated to enhance the disposition of individuals with depression. The supplement was not viewed as protection for the brain, and was expelled from the production. Nonetheless, you can guarantee your mind gets a standard supply of tryptophan by including no less than one portion of protein at every dinner ie. Meat, fish, eggs, milk, cheddar, nuts, beans, lentils (dhal), or meat substitute, for example, textured vegetable protein.

Eat a wide assortment of foods to keep your diet intriguing, and to guarantee you get all the micronutrients you require. If you have bread at one meal, try to switch to oaks, or potatoes, rice, or sweet potatoes at the other. Make sure you incorporate no less than 2 servings of leafy foods/vegetables, and a protein food at every meal.

# Chapter 5

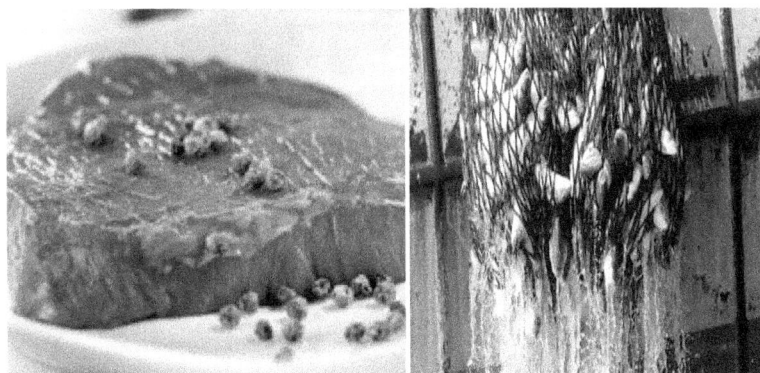

## RED MEAT AND FISH

Incorporate some red meat and fish, because they have a great amount of vitamin B12, another supplement that supports your state of mind. If you are vegan, or have a restricted dietary plan, incorporate soy meat and yeast to expand your intake of this vitamin. Incorporate fish, particularly sleek fish, in your diet. A study proposes that omega 3 oil supplements may reduce side effects in individuals with depression. An equalization of omega 3 and omega 6 oils in your diet is essential.

1. Include more omega 3-rich wild fish -incorporate 2-4 servings a week (2 servings if you are pregnant or breastfeeding). If you are purchasing fish in a can, pick fish canned in water, saline solution or tomato sauce as opposed to in sunflower oil (this is high in omega 6).

2. If you deep fry food utilize oil high in monounsaturated fat. Olive or Grape seed oil.

3. Choose monounsaturated margarine or spread. Keep away from margarines or low fat spreads containing

omega 6 polyunsaturated, or hydrogenated trans fats (trans fats are harming in developing a health state of mind.)

4. Avoid processed foods, for example, pies, hotdogs, and cakes-these are high in trans-fat.

If you don't care for fish you could try an omega 3 supplement (pick one that is cleansed, contain no vitamins and has a high eicosapenanoic corrosive (EPA) content-take 1g each day). If you are a veggie lover, try a flax seed supplement.

# Chapter 6

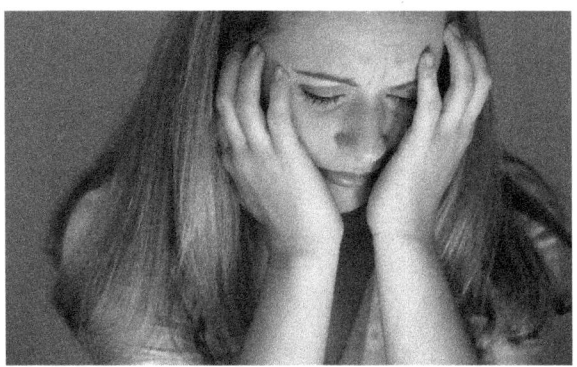

## DEPRESSION AND DIET

Depression influences individual's in various ways. Some individuals lose interest in food, or can't persuade themselves to go shopping or cook. Others discover they need to eat more and put on weight when they are miserable. Some medications can also expand or reduce your hunger-if you are worried your prescription you are taking has accelerated your weight address this issue with your doctor.

Unreasonable weight reduction or weight addition can make your depression worse. Weight reduction and absence of good nourishment will deny the mind of glucose, and alternate supplements that control disposition-you may require the help of a dietitian to overcome this issue.

If you are overweight get guidance from your dietitian to help you develop a healthier eating habit, and be cautious on how much fat and sugar you allow in your diet (no fries, pies, cakes, puddings, desserts, chocolate, or sweet beverages), utilize less fat in cooking, less liquor consumption, maintain your distance from sugary beverages, and increase the time you spend working out.

# Chapter 7

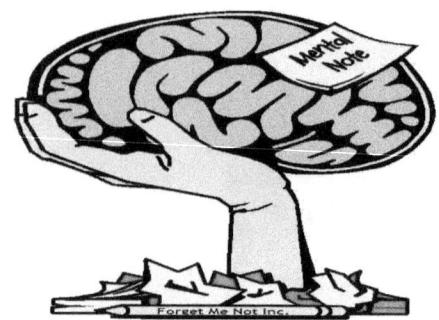

## CONCENTRATION AND MEMORY

Studies has shown blueberries help "concentration and memory" for up to five hours. Blueberries also contain a "cocktail of antioxidants including anthocyanins, proanthocyanidins, reseratrol, and tannis", research shows they support focus, and protect against cancer, coronary illness, and dimensia. Green tea helps you focus for two reasons: one, it contains caffeine, and two, it contains l'theanine. The caffeine helps you focus and enhances your sharpness.

Well, what is l'theanine? It's a ingredient that "expand alpha-wave action", which discharges caffeine more gradually, which can discharge your crashing. The two additionally joins to "create a better capacity to focus attention, with change of both rate and accuracy". If you handle the caffeine well, bringing green tea into your diet it's virtually an easy decision.

Not sufficiently drinking fluid has huge ramifications for mental health. The early impacts of dehydration can influence our emotions and conduct. An adult lose more or less than 2.5

liters of water every day through the lungs as water vapor, through the skin as sweat, and through the kidneys as urine. If you don't drink enough fluids to replace this output then you can experience side effects of dehydration, including crankiness, loss of concentration that can reduce your mental capacity.

Espresso, colas, some caffeinated drinks and tea all contain caffeine, which some individuals utilization to support their energy levels. A large amount of caffeine can increase pulse, nervousness, depression and sleeplessness. Caffeine additionally has a diuretic impact in the body. Consequently you should not depend on caffeine-based fluids.

If you do buy drinks with caffeine in them, try to restrict yourself to only 3-4 cups every day and drink different fluids, for example water, natural fruit or vegetable juice, and non-stimulant teas. Chocolate also contains caffeine, and should be limited as a treat.

# Chapter 8

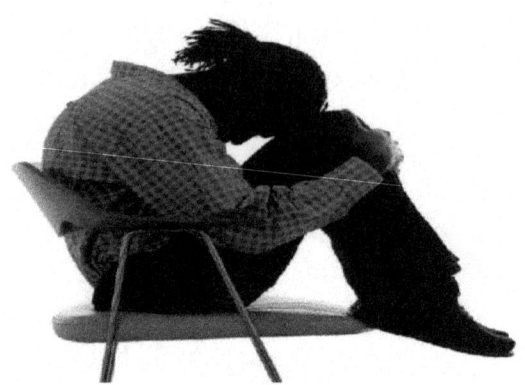

## LIMITS AND TRIGGERS

Limit your liquor intake. Liquor has a depressive impact on the brain and can bring down your temperament. It is also a toxin that must be detoxified by the liver; but for this the body utilizes thiamin, zinc and different supplements -this can drain your reserves, particularly if your diet is poor. Thiamin and other vitamin deficiencies are common in heavy drinkers, and can lead to a low temperament, crankiness and/ or forceful conduct, and mental health issues. Since the body utilizes essential supplements to process liquor, individuals who experience depression should consider staying away from liquor until they have recovered. And even then, in light of liquor's depressant impacts, you should consider drinking just small amounts once every week. The prescribed safe cutoff point for liquor is two units a day for women, and three units for men.

### WORKING OUT

Working out triggers endorphins-chemicals that trigger "happiness" in the brain, that help us to unwind and feel cheerful.  Exercise is especially essential for individuals with depression, because it also gives structure and reason to the day.  Outdoor practice that opens us to daylight is particularly important as it influences the pineal gland and helps temperament.

Working out is helps too if you are attempting to control your weight.  The more you work out, the less you have to eliminate your caloric intake to control your weight.  It is also helpful for heart health, and it guarantees you will build muscle, building a healthier conditioned body.  It also eliminates bone mass problems, and the danger of osteoporosis.

Walking is the least demanding, least expensive and best type of activity.  Swimming is useful for individuals with joint issues who can't do the activities at the gym.  Cycling is also a great way to exercise.  Whatever activity you choose, begins with 20 minutes no less than three times each week, and expand this as your wellness moves forward.

# Chapter 9

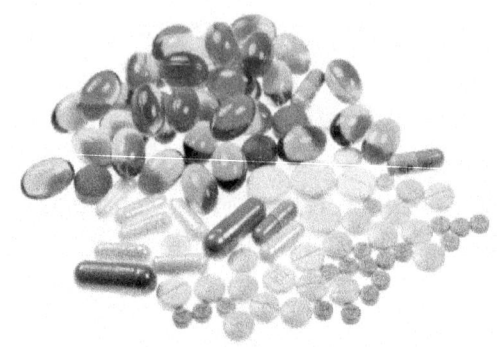

## DIETARY SUPPLEMENTS

Dietary supplements are an important part of your process towards developing your mental health through a good diet. Consider these tips to aid in the cause.

1. Choose a one-a-day multivitamin containing the full prescribed day by day intake of every vitamin and mineral. These items are protected because they don't contain unnecessary measures of any single supplement (however you should avoid supplements containing vitamin A as it is harmful in high dosages)

2. If your specialist supports vitamins or minerals for you, let him /her know about any medications you are taking.

3. If you do take a multivitamin supplement, avoid eating liver and other offal items, for example, pate, as these are additionally high in vitamin A.

It is vital to remember supplements are not a substitute for a healthy diet, and you should keep up a diverse and adjusted diet. Various studies have connected the intake of some supplements with depression. Complex starches and some food segments, for example, folic corrosive, omega-3 unsaturated fats, selenium and tryptophan in supplement form, are said to cause depression.

People with low intakes of foliate, or folic corrosive, are more likely to develop depression more than those with higher intakes. Most people struggle with eating a good diet and taking dietary supplements. Exercising seems to have become a rare practice among modern man. If your aim is to achieve good mental health through your diet, including good food and good food habits; it is very importance that you stick to the procedure explained in this book. With good healthy diet and exercise, you can reach your goal of gaining good mental health.

# Conclusion

Thank you again for choosing this book!

I hope this book was able to help you begin your journey eating with your mental health in mind.

The next step is to start with small changes, and work your way to your goal.

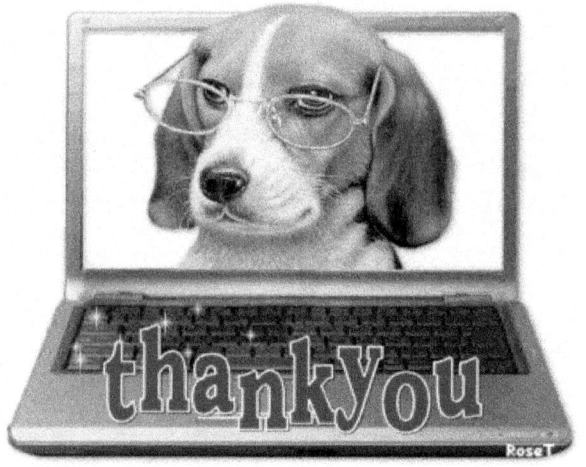

Finally, if you enjoyed this book would you be kind enough to leave a review for this book on Amazon?    It'd be greatly appreciated!

Leave a review for this book on Amazon.com!

Thank you and good luck!

# Preview of 'JUICING TO HELP MENTAL ILLNESS'

Mental illness is becoming more and more common in today's world, and most of the times unrecognized, the cause of this may be simple nutrient deficiency. If not addressed, mental illnesses cause by nutrient deficiency can take a serious toll on our physical and mental health, which is why it is important to correct it early through juicing and other nutritional means.

Most people don't know that many chronic and mental illnesses are a direct result of nutrient deficiencies, which can be easily and quickly remedied through juicing.

## Chapter 1
### *BERRY A-PEELING*

*INGREDIENTS*

*APPLES-2 LARGE (3-1/4" DIA)*

*LIME-1/2 FRUIT (2" DIA)*

*STRAWBERRIES-3 CUP, WHOLE*

*DIRECTIONS: PROCESS ALL INGREDIENTS IN A JUICER, SHAKER OR STIR AND SERVE*

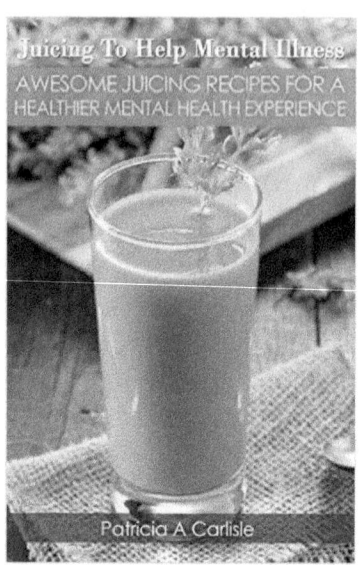

go to: amazon.com to check out the rest of the book!

# Check Out My Other Books

Below you'll find some of my other popular books that are popular on Amazon and Kindle. Alternatively, you can visit my author page on Amazon to see other work done by me.

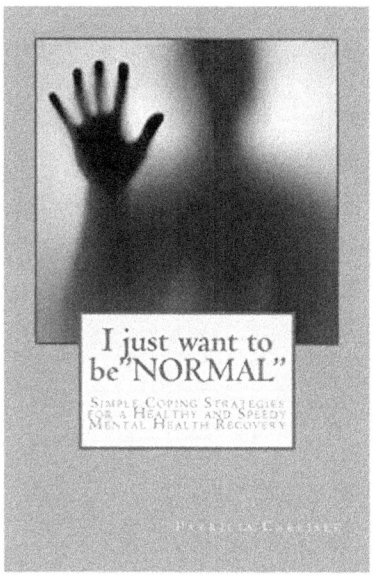

**I just want to be "NORMAL" Simple Coping Strategies for a Healthy and Spcedy Mental Health Recovery.**

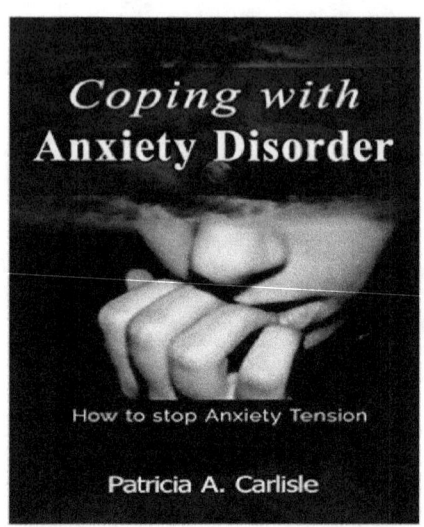

**Coping with Anxiety Disorder: How to stop Anxiety Tension.**

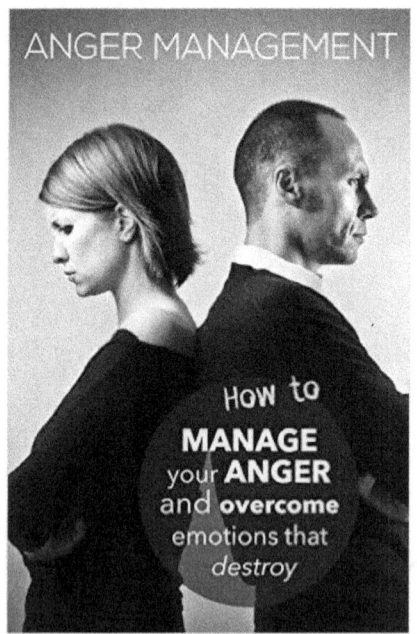

**Anger Management: How to manage your anger and overcome emotions that destroy.**

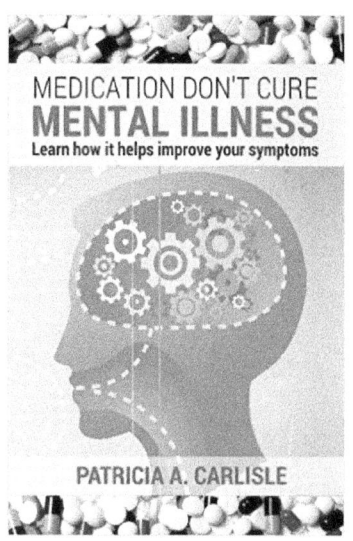

Medication don't cure mental illness:  Learn how it helps improve your symptoms.

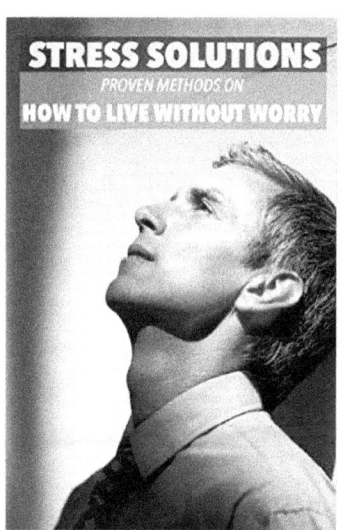

Stress Solutions:  Proven methods on how to live without worry.

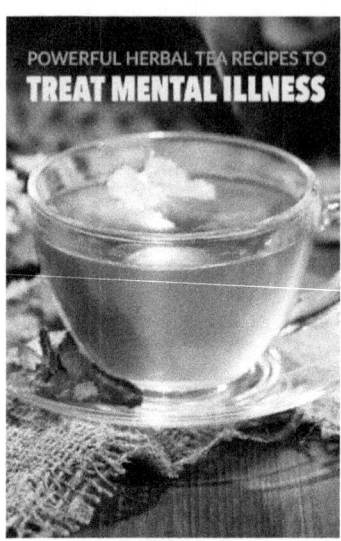

**Powerful herbal recipes to treat Mental Illness.**

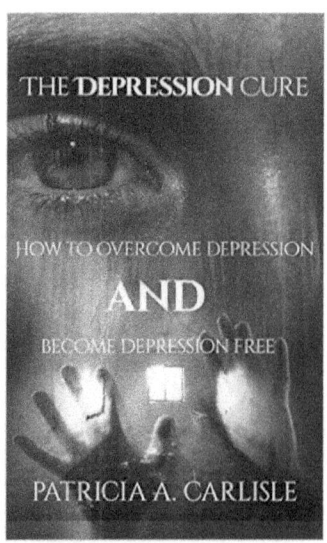

**The Depression Cure: How to overcome depression and become depression free.**

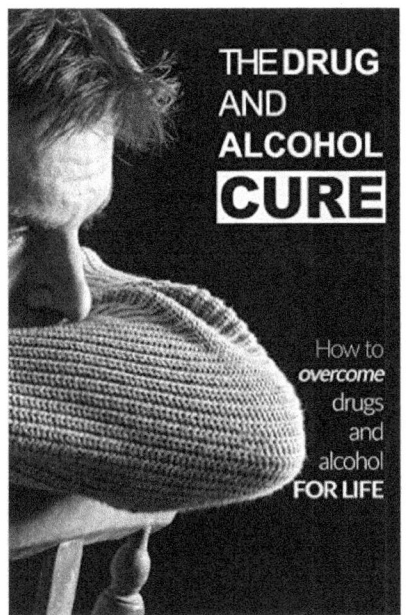

**The Drug and Alcohol Cure: How to overcome drugs and alcohol for life.**

You can simply search for these titles on the Amazon website.

# BONUS: SUBSCRIBE TO THE FREE BOOK

## Beginners Guide to Yoga & Meditation

"Stressed out? Do You Feel Like The World Is Crashing Down Around You? Want To Take A Vacation That Will Relax Your Mind, Body And Spirit? Well this Easy To Read Step By Step

E-Book Makes It All Possible!"

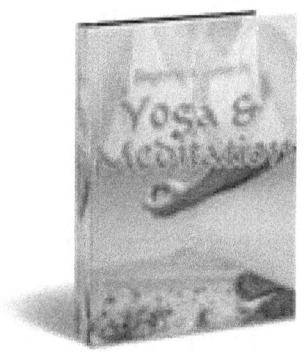

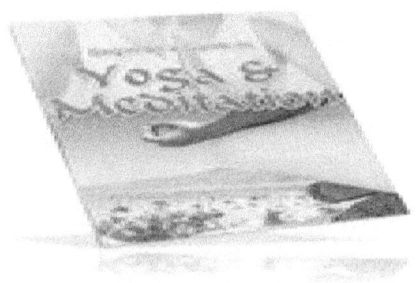

Instructions on how to join our mailing list, and receive a free copy of "Yoga and Meditation" can be found in any of my Kindle eBooks.

# NOTES

# NOTE

# NOTE

# NOTE

# NOTES

# NOTES

www.ingramcontent.com/pod-product-compliance
Lightning Source LLC
Chambersburg PA
CBHW070230210526
45168CB00019B/1471